DRUG
DANGERS

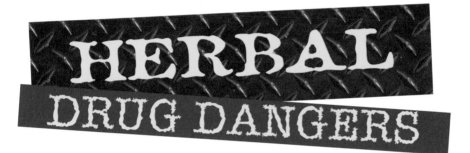

Judy Monroe

Enslow Publishers, Inc.

40 Industrial Road	PO Box 38
Box 398	Aldershot
Berkeley Heights, NJ 07922	Hants GU12 6BP
USA	UK

http://www.enslow.com

Library of Congress Cataloging-in-Publication Data

Monroe, Judy.
    Herbal drug dangers / Judy Monroe
        p. cm. — (Drug dangers)
    Includes bibliographical references and index.
    Summary: Discusses the use of "herbal drugs" and some of their
possible dangers.
    ISBN 0-7660-1319-7
    1. Herbs—Toxicology—Juvenile literature. 2. Materia medica,
Vegetable—Toxicology—Juvenile literature. 3. Herbs—Therapeutic use—
Juvenile literature. [1. Herbs. 2. Drug abuse.] I. Title. II. Series.

RA1250.M66   2000
615.9'52—dc21   99-038290

Printed in the United States of America

10 9 8 7 6 5 4 3 2 1

To Our Readers:
All Internet addresses in this book were active and appropriate when we
went to press. Any comments or suggestions can be sent by e-mail to
Comments@enslow.com or to the address on the back cover.

Photo Credits: © Steven Foster, pp. 11, 18, 22, 27, 33, 34, 37, 38, 39, 41, 49.

Cover Photo: All images, © Steven Foster

contents

Titles in the **Drug Dangers** series:

Alcohol Drug Dangers
ISBN 0-7660-1159-3

Amphetamine Drug Dangers
ISBN 0-7660-1321-9

Crack and Cocaine Drug Dangers
ISBN 0-7660-1155-0

Diet Pill Drug Dangers
ISBN 0-7660-1158-5

Ecstasy and Other Designer Drug Dangers
ISBN 0-7660-1322-7

Herbal Drug Dangers
ISBN 0-7660-1319-7

Heroin Drug Dangers
ISBN 0-7660-1156-9

Inhalant Drug Dangers
ISBN 0-7660-1153-4

LSD, PCP, and Hallucinogen Drug Dangers
ISBN 0-7660-1318-9

Marijuana Drug Dangers
ISBN 0-7660-1214-X

Speed and Methamphetamine Drug Dangers
ISBN 0-7660-1157-7

Steroid Drug Dangers
ISBN 0-7660-1154-2

Tobacco and Nicotine Drug Dangers
ISBN 0-7660-1317-0

Tranquilizer, Barbiturate, and Downer
Drug Dangers
ISBN 0-7660-1320-0

one

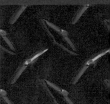

Pete's Story

Early in March 1996, Pete, age twenty, finished his exams. Pete was a senior at the State University of New York at Albany. He was studying history and theater.

After making plans for how to spend his spring break, he telephoned his parents. He told them he was going to Panama City, Florida, with several friends. He was going to have fun during his vacation. That was the last time Pete ever talked to his parents.

Just a few days later, at 6:00 P.M. on March 7, Pete's parents got a telephone call at their home in Long Island, New York. The police asked if they could come over. The officers had something to tell them.

"For two or three minutes, I didn't think anything of it," remembered Pete's mom. "Then

5

my blood just went cold as ice and I said, 'Oh, my God, I hope it's not Pete.'"[1]

But the police officer had bad news. "I'm sorry to have to tell you this. Your son is dead," he told the parents.[2]

What had caused Pete's death? Pete's mom talked to some of the friends with whom Pete had been on vacation, and found the answer. During the day on March 6, Pete and his friends wandered in and out of Panama City's small shops along the beach. They saw flashy signs and posters. Many advertised herbal supplements with names like Cloud 9™, Herbal Ecstacy™ (sic), and Ultimate Xphoria™. Pamphlets that came with these herbs said they were natural and legal—and that the pills gave users a safe high.

That evening, Pete and his friends took Ultimate Xphoria. The package instructions said to take four tablets. The store clerk, though, recommended twelve to fifteen tablets. Pete took eight. Soon he complained of a tingling sensation and a headache. When his friends went out for the evening, Pete stayed at the motel.[3]

Later that evening, when Pete's friends returned to the motel, they found him lying on the floor. He was dead. The friends then called the police. According to the report of the local medical examiner, Pete had overdosed on the herbs in Ultimate Xphoria.[4]

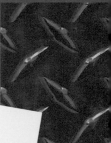

two

Social

Issues

Herbal remedies are a big and rapidly growing business. Millions of people buy and take them. But herbal remedies are not as closely regulated (controlled by laws) as are prescription drugs. This lack of regulation has created health problems— sometimes deadly—for many who take these products.

Who Takes Them—and Why?

Surveys show that more than half of American adults use herbal remedies.[1] Most doctors in the United States, however, know little about herbals, and rarely recommend them to patients. In addition, most herbal remedies are not covered by health insurance. As of 1997, just twelve American pharmacy schools had courses on the use of herbal remedies.[2] Few medical doctors receive training in prescribing herbals or in using herbals as part of a treatment plan.

Herbal medicine is much more accepted by consumers and doctors in Europe than by people in the United States. In Germany, for example:

- six hundred to seven hundred plant-based remedies are for sale;[3]

- many German doctors prescribe herbal medicines; and[4]

- many herbal remedies are accepted by the government's health insurance.[5]

If doctors in the United States are not recommending or prescribing herbal remedies, why are people using them? Some people take them to try to prevent health problems from developing. Some want to maintain their current health by using herbals. One owner of a health food store said that her customers "see herbs as a good way to strengthen the immune system to keep from getting sick in the first place."[6]

Other people take herbal remedies because herbals sometimes cost less than other medicines. It is also easy to find and buy them. A wide variety of herbal remedies are available through mail-order catalogs, through the Internet, and in all kinds of local stores: supermarkets, health food stores, drugstores, and convenience stores. The bottom line is that people want more control over their own health care.[7] Herb-based remedies seem like one way to achieve this control. People can buy and take them without having to see a doctor or other health care professional. But this is not always a good thing.

People are also turning to herbal remedies because they believe natural is better.[8] Many people believe that because herbals are natural, they must be safe. This is not always true. Just because something is natural does not mean it is good for you or that it will not harm you. Arsenic and hemlock are natural, but both are strong, potentially deadly poisons.

The "natural is better" belief goes along with America's back-to-nature quest. Since the 1970s, Americans have increasingly turned to natural products. Many people look for and buy natural foods and beverages, and clothing made from natural fibers. This back-to-nature movement, combined with Americans' desire to be healthy, has resulted in growing interest in herbal remedies.[9]

Also, some people (like Pete from Chapter 1) take herbs as a substitute for illegal drugs. Some herbal products claim to boost energy or give users a natural high.

Booming Business

Before the 1970s, people often had to look hard to find herbal remedies. Today, these products are easy to find. They are sold in many different stores and are widely available. This is good news for those in the herbal business.

"Everybody I know that's in the herb business is booming," says Ed Smith, owner of Herb Pharm, an Oregon-based herbal products company. "The whole self-care industry is booming, whether it's weight-loss tablets, herbs or vitamins and minerals. And a lot of the stuff that's very, very popular today was considered 'fringe' twenty years ago. It's becoming very mainstream."[10]

Smith is right. Herbal supplements are some of the hottest selling items today. Some numbers from Packaged Facts, a market research company in New York City are shown on the next page.

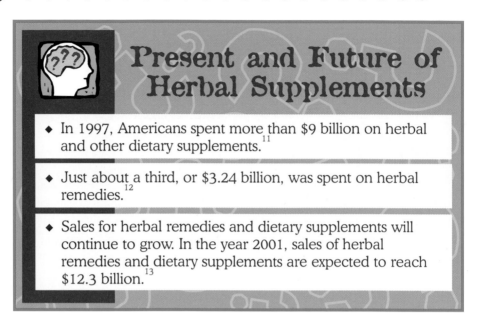

Present and Future of Herbal Supplements

- In 1997, Americans spent more than $9 billion on herbal and other dietary supplements.[11]

- Just about a third, or $3.24 billion, was spent on herbal remedies.[12]

- Sales for herbal remedies and dietary supplements will continue to grow. In the year 2001, sales of herbal remedies and dietary supplements are expected to reach $12.3 billion.[13]

Does Natural Mean Safe?

Herbal remedies contain substances that can have powerful effects on the mind or body, so herbal remedies can be dangerous. Roseanne Philen knows this is true. Philen is a scientist at the Centers for Disease Control (CDC) in Atlanta, Georgia. Her job is to find out why people get sick. Sometimes herbs have caused people to become ill or even die.

She has found that the wrong herb can get into a remedy. Workers who pick herb plants do not always know much about the herb. Sometimes they collect the poisonous parts of an herb. Or they pick the wrong plant.

In 1994, seven people in New York City became ill. The culprit was an herbal tea. The tea was made from a poisonous plant. The people who drank the poisoned tea soon developed rapid heartbeat, fever, and red skin. Three were rushed to hospitals for emergency treatment. Luckily, all recovered.

Chaparral is an herb that comes from a shrub that grows in the Southwest. People take it for its supposed cancer-curing and blood-purifying properties. It can cause serious liver damage. One sixty-year-old woman took chaparral capsules for ten months. She developed stomach pain, loss of appetite, and yellowish skin. She was rushed to the hospital. What had happened? The chaparral had damaged her liver so badly that she needed a transplant. Luckily, the transplant worked, and she recovered.[14]

People who sell herbs may not know much about their products. They may not be aware of the potential for harm that herbs or excess amounts of herbs can cause. One example of product ignorance was the clerk

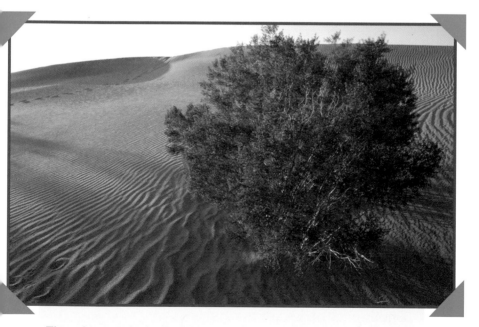

The chaparral shrub grows in the southwestern part of the United States. Chaparral is said to have cancer-curing and blood purifying properties. It can, however, cause liver damage.

The Two Types of Medicines in the United States

Prescription	Medicines that can be sold only with the written instruction of a licensed medical doctor.
Nonprescription or Over-the-counter (OTC)	Medicines that can be bought and used without a doctor's supervision.

What Medicines Are Used For

Medicines Can	Examples
Prevent Diseases	Vaccines for polio
Fight germs that cause disease	Penicillin and other antibiotics
Relieve physical pain	Aspirin and aspirin substitutes
Treat specific health problems or conditions	Medicine for blood pressure or allergies

from Chapter 1 who told Pete and his friends to take more Ultimate Xphoria than the package instructions recommended.

Comparing Medicines and Herbal Remedies

Many people think that herbal remedies are tested and approved by the federal government.[15] This is not true. In the United States, herbal remedies seldom go through any scientific testing and the approval process is not as strict as it is for prescription drugs.

Unlike herbal remedies, prescription and over-the-counter (OTC) nonprescription medicines have undergone ten to twenty years of careful testing. These tests must prove that these medicines are safe and effective (work for certain uses). Companies spend millions of dollars to make sure their medicines meet federal laws for safety and effectiveness. In fact, the companies must prove to the government that their products work safely when used as directed.

The Law

The Food and Drug Administration (FDA) regulates medicines and foods. Until the early 1990s, the FDA regulated other products, such as vitamins, minerals, and herbs. Then Congress passed The Dietary Supplement and Health Education Act (DSHEA) of 1994.

This law created a new category of products—dietary supplements—separate from food or drugs. In passing DSHEA, Congress recognized that:

◆ many people believe dietary supplements offer health benefits; and

◆ people want a greater opportunity to determine whether supplements may help them.[16]

The DSHEA gives makers of vitamins, minerals, and herbal remedies much more freedom to make, market (promote), and sell their products. Companies do not have to prove that their herbal products are safe or that they work.

The DSHEA greatly limits the FDA's power over herbal products. The FDA has little control over the manufacture, promotion, and selling of herbal products. For example, before the FDA can stop the sale of an herbal product, it must prove that taking the product is dangerous or very risky. The process of gathering this proof takes a long time and a great deal of money.

Labeling and Advertising

According to the FDA, a company cannot claim that an herbal remedy cures, treats, or prevents a disease or illness. The FDA recently sent a warning letter to one company. This company claimed its herbal remedy "may be beneficial for . . . psoriasis."[17] Psoriasis is a chronic skin disease. People with psoriasis often have red, scaly, itchy patches on their skin.

Under the DSHEA, if companies make claims, then the claim or herbal label must carry this warning:

> This statement has not been evaluated by the Food and Drug Administration. This product is not intended to diagnose, treat, cure, or prevent any disease.

Even with this warning, many people mistakenly assume that herbal remedies are FDA-approved and safe.[18]

Under the DSHEA, President Bill Clinton formed the Commission on Dietary Supplement Labels (CDSL) in 1995. In November 1997, the CDSL published an important report. In part, the CDSL report:

- ◆ encourages scientific studies to identify if dietary supplements affect health and diseases;

- ◆ recommends that the FDA stop the sale of a product if it seems unsafe; and

- ◆ recommends that the FDA and the companies work together to develop warning statements on dietary-supplement labels.

Based on the CDSL report, the FDA proposed making

rules for claims and labels of dietary supplements. These changes will make claims and labels more reliable and uniform. Here are two highlights from the April 1998 FDA proposal.

◆ If a claim states or implies that a product treats, cures, or prevents health conditions, the FDA will consider it a medicine. The company must then follow the same laws as for prescription and over-the-counter drugs.

◆ Companies will need to follow the FDA's new rules for Dietary Supplement Labels.

The Federal Trade Commission (FTC) regulates advertising for dietary supplements and most other products sold to consumers. The FDA works closely with the FTC in this area. However, the Food and Drug Administration's work is directed by different laws.

Safety Concerns

In 1996, some five hundred serious complications from various dietary supplements, including herbs, were reported to the FDA.[20] This number probably does not reflect all problems associated with herbals, however. The problem is that no one is tracking bad reactions to herbal remedies, and many problems may go unreported or unnoticed.

There is another safety concern with herbal remedies. If a prescription or over-the-counter medicine has caused people serious harm, the FDA can stop its sales. But if an herbal product has harmed people, the FDA may or may not be able to pull it off store shelves.

The FDA gets information about herbal products very slowly. Before the FDA can react, it must first wait for reports from doctors, hospitals, health agencies, or individuals. Reports can take months to arrive at the FDA. Then FDA officials must track the information for a while to see if a pattern develops.

The lack of information about many herbal supplements is another problem for the FDA. Companies that make herbals may not have much information on their products. In contrast, companies that make prescription and over-the-counter medicines can tell the FDA:

- ◆ exactly what is in their medicine;

- ◆ how much is prescribed;

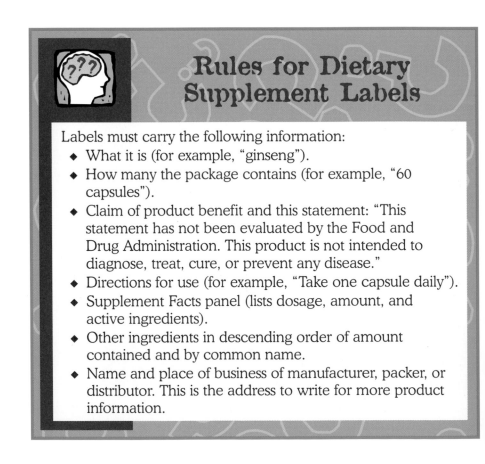

Rules for Dietary Supplement Labels

Labels must carry the following information:
- ◆ What it is (for example, "ginseng").
- ◆ How many the package contains (for example, "60 capsules").
- ◆ Claim of product benefit and this statement: "This statement has not been evaluated by the Food and Drug Administration. This product is not intended to diagnose, treat, cure, or prevent any disease."
- ◆ Directions for use (for example, "Take one capsule daily").
- ◆ Supplement Facts panel (lists dosage, amount, and active ingredients).
- ◆ Other ingredients in descending order of amount contained and by common name.
- ◆ Name and place of business of manufacturer, packer, or distributor. This is the address to write for more product information.

◆ the safe dosage (amount to take); and

◆ what side (bad) effects have shown up in years of testing.

Both the Centers for Disease Control (CDC) and the American Association of Poison Control Centers help the FDA track problems with medicines. But they have no good way to track problems with herbal supplements.

In addition to the FDA, individual states can also restrict or stop the sale of harmful herbal remedies. Georgia has identified yohimbe as a dangerous drug. Yohimbe makers claim it stops chest pain and impotence. As a result of the dangers identified with its use, however, this herb can only be sold by prescription. Florida has stopped the sale of all ephedra-containing products. Ephedra is used to unclog nasal passages. It also speeds up the heart rate and increases blood pressure. Several other states have restricted its sales. Ephedra, also known as ma huang, has caused serious health problems.

Self-Regulation

So far, the herbal-supplement industry has not done a very good job of regulating, or controlling, itself.[21] For example, the American Herbal Products Association (AHPA) asked its members to stop selling chaparral, an herb that can cause serious liver problems. It then suggested that the labels on chaparral bottles include strong cautions and a hot line (a toll-free phone number) to report problems. The AHPA also recommended that comfrey be sold for external (topical) use only, rather than prohibiting its sale entirely. Like chaparral, comfrey is a dangerous herb that is reported to heal broken bones, ulcers, and burns, and to stop internal bleeding.

Consumer Reports magazine checked the labels on the bottles of both herbs. They found chaparral bottles that carried a "lukewarm warning and no hotline number."[22] They also "found comfrey—in capsules, for internal use."[23]

Furthermore, the herbal industry seldom enforces quality control among its products. Several studies have found that herbal remedies often vary greatly in the quality and quantity of herbs they contain and what part of the herb is used. (Only specific parts of any herb contain active ingredients.)

What Is In That Pill, Tablet, or Capsule?

Since herbal supplements are not being as carefully regulated as prescription and over-the-counter

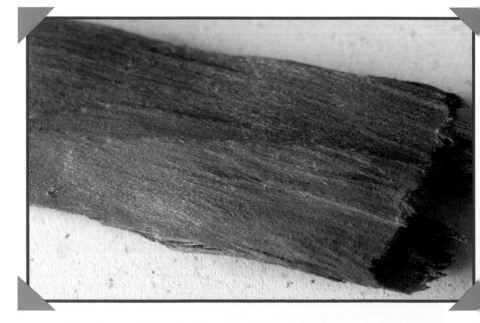

The state of Georgia has identified yohimbe as a dangerous substance. As a result, the herb is now sold only by prescription.

medications, just what are consumers getting? Due to the lack of standards, consumers have no way to be sure:

◆ whether an herbal remedy's ingredients are in a form the body can use. Companies may use whole plants or plant parts, cut pieces or finely ground pieces.

◆ whether an herb in one bottle is as potent, or strong, as the same herb in another bottle. Each herb plant can vary a lot in its strength. Growing conditions, handling, and storage also affect the herb's strength.

◆ what exactly is in an herbal remedy.

◆ if the dosage is correct, too much, or too little.

◆ whether the next bottle of an herbal by the same or a different company will have the same ingredients.

◆ whether the herbs and other ingredients were stored correctly. Heat, light, and moisture can affect herbs and other ingredients.

◆ whether an herbal remedy is safe.

In 1995, *Consumer Reports* magazine tested ten brands of ginseng. This Asian root has been a popular herbal for many years. It supposedly increases energy levels, improves the appetite and breathing, and stimulates the immune system. *Consumer Reports* "found a wide variation, from brand to brand. . . . Some pills had 10 or 20 times as much others, and one brand had very little ginsenoside [the active ingredient in ginseng]."[24]

Other tests published in a medical journal came up with the same results. In fact, a few so-called ginseng products actually contained no ginseng at all.[25] In another study, fifty-four ginseng products were tested. One quarter, or 25 percent, contained no ginseng.

Selling Harmful Herbals

The herb ephedra, also called ma huang, accounts for many complaints to the FDA. It has caused a number of deaths. The FDA and medical researchers have also identified other dangerous herbs.

In 1992, the FDA warned companies to stop selling herbal remedies with gum guar. Gum guar swells once ingested, causing people to feel full, and making it easier to lose weight. A number of people developed serious swallowing problems from taking these products. One person died.

At least seventeen people developed liver disease from taking chaparral.[26] For now, the FDA has sent out a warning about using the herb. Many companies have stopped making products with chaparral. However, consumers can still buy this herb at stores across the country.

Lack of Reliable Information

Most herbals are marketed, or promoted, based on anecdotes—word of mouth. People may say that an herbal remedy has helped them, but word-of-mouth descriptions are not always the most reliable or accurate type of information. There is no way to tell for sure whether an herbal remedy was effective or whether the person taking it would have eventually achieved the desired result without the use of herbals. Many illnesses clear up on their own, no matter what someone takes to help the healing process.

Also, people sometimes feel better simply because they *think* they have taken a remedy—even if what they have taken is a sugar pill with no active ingredients. This phenomenon is known as the placebo effect.

Finding accurate, reliable information about the benefits and risks of herbal remedies can be difficult. Most scientific studies have been done in Europe, especially Germany. But Germany does not demand the same level of scientific evidence that the United States does. Nonetheless, American and British researchers have begun to translate and review these German studies.

Studies of some herbal supplements are now under way in the United States. The Office of Alternative Medicine (OAM) in Washington, D.C., is running studies on a handful of herbal remedies. Congress created OAM in 1992. It is part of the National Institutes of Health. It will take time, though, to run the studies and analyze the results.

Ask an Expert?

Some people ask health-food store workers for herbal advice. Is that a good idea? In 1993, the FDA sent staff members undercover to health-food stores across America. Some asked for help for problems with their immune systems. The immune system helps the body fight off diseases. Others asked for something to reduce high blood pressure or to deal with cancer.

In all, they asked 129 times. They got specific recommendations 120 times from various clerks. The advice ranged from honeysuckle crystals, shark cartilage, and garlic to saw palmetto. The bottom line—health-food clerks are not always experts in herbal remedies.

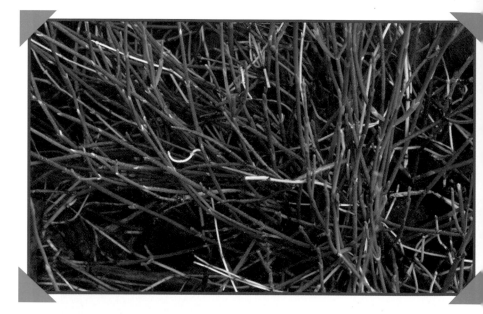

The herb known as ephedra or ma huang has been identified as a dangerous substance. It accounts for many complaints to the Food and Drug Administration, and has caused a number of deaths nationwide.

Pharmacists may give advice about herbal remedies. But many have no training on herbals. In one study, *Consumer Reports* asked pharmacists about various herbs. They got confusing answers and even wrong information. One pharmacist said, "If it's sold over the counter, it's FDA approved."[27] The pharmacist was wrong. Herbal supplements are sold over the counter but they are *not* always FDA-approved.

The American Council on Pharmaceutical Education (ACPE) has asked pharmacists to be careful when telling people about herbals. ACPE provides educational classes for pharmacists, and warns that "The majority of popular claims associated with herbal products are probably either false or unproved."[28]

three

Real-Life Examples of Herbal Abuse

A young nursing student went to see her physician, Dr. Clair Eliason. The young student said she had been losing weight for no reason. She was also edgy and nervous and no longer menstruated every month. Based on her symptoms, said Dr. Eliason, the young woman appeared to have an overactive thyroid gland. The thyroid is located in front of and to both sides of the windpipe. It produces the hormone thyroxin. Thyroxine controls metabolism, or how the body breaks down and uses food.

Dangerous Thyroid Supplement

Dr. Eliason found instead that the young woman was taking an herbal supplement that contained about four or five times the recommended dosage of thyroid tissue. This substance is in prescription thyroid-replacement medicines.

Said Dr. Eliason, "This woman had no idea what she was taking. She said she had been feeling tired, and this supplement was recommended to her by the clerk in the health-food store. I was amazed they were allowed to sell this—the same medication that requires a prescription from a doctor was being sold over the counter."[1]

Case of Contamination

A young woman took an herbal laxative that was supposed to contain the herb plantain. A laxative helps produce bowel movements. The woman's heart rate became abnormal, and she had a heart attack. The FDA quickly issued warnings about supplements with plantain. However, the FDA soon learned that the supplement she took was actually contaminated. It contained the wrong herb.

When the FDA tested the supplement, they did not find any plantain. Instead, they found digitalis. This powerful herb is used in prescription medicines for the heart. If too much digitalis is taken, a person can vomit, get dizzy, and have bad headaches. They can also have a heart attack.[2]

The Agony of Herbal Drugs

Valerie had never tried Herbal Ecstacy (sic). In fact, the sixteen-year-old was a vegetarian and a competitive swimmer. She did not take drugs, smoke, or drink alcoholic beverages. In the summer of 1994, Valerie and a friend went to see Hole, a favorite band. She noticed a lot of teens at a nearby booth that advertised Herbal Ecstacy (sic).

Neither Valerie nor her friend knew what Herbal Ecstacy (sic) was. "The vendor told us these little blue pills were a safe, all-natural energy source with no side effects and that we needed to take a lot. I was tired and Hole wasn't going to play for another five hours. I thought it might help to wake me up."[3]

The vendor suggested Valerie take ten pills. For her larger friend, the vendor recommended fifteen. Valerie took ten pills. Within thirty minutes, her heart began to pound wildly. She fainted three times. Her friend became very sick. Both were rushed to a hospital emergency room and had their stomachs pumped. "They told us we almost died," said Valerie.[4]

Ill from Mandrake

In 1997, a thirty-one-year-old man bought four small packages of an herb root called mandrake at a local health-food store. He said he tried the herb because, "It's a brain drug. It increases oxygen to the brain."[5]

He mixed all four packages into a glass of milk. Then he drank the milk and root bits. Several hours later, he began vomiting continually and felt very nauseated. He was rushed to a hospital emergency room. After a night in the hospital, he felt fine. His nausea and vomiting had stopped, and he had no other bad effects.

Doctors at the hospital bought the same packages at the same health-food store. They tested the herb and did some research. They found that there are two versions of mandrake. The man who got so sick thought he had taken *Mandrogora officinarum*, known as mandrake.[6] This herb can cause people to get high and have hallucinations—imaginary sights, sounds, and feelings.

What the man really took was *Podophyllum pelatum*. This herb is also known as mandrake, but this version is a strong and unpredictable laxative.

The doctors who treated this man found another case of mistaken mandrake. They read an account posted to the Usenet newsgroup <http://www.alt.drugs> on the World Wide Web. This person wrote,

> I decided to experiment with mandrake root. These drugs are known to cause some unpleasant (but, I thought, hallucinogenic) effects. I made tea with around 6 tablespoons of mandrake, drank a bunch, nothing, drank another glass and went out for dinner. As soon as I ate a meal, my stomach began to hurt . . . that feeling turned into the most horrific drug experience I can imagine.[7]

This person had continual vomiting and diarrhea. He was sick for about ten hours. Then he felt better, with no other side effects. The doctors said, "We believe this person also mistakenly took the wrong version of mandrake."[8]

Herbal Tea Makes Woman Sick

In the early 1990s, Randi was having trouble with constipation. She was not able to have regular bowel movements. She asked a friend for advice. "My friend suggested I try this herbal tea that everyone was talking about," said Randi.[9] Although some women supposedly lost weight on it, her friend told her most take it to stop constipation.

Randi read the list of ingredients on the label of the herbal tea. "I wanted to be sure it didn't contain any laxatives. I was trying to keep away from those because I know how dangerous they can be."[10] She spotted some Latin names of ingredients that she did not know. But she decided not to be concerned. "I figured it was just an herbal tea. It wouldn't do me any harm."[11]

She began drinking two cups a day. She followed the directions on the box to make her daily tea. The herbal tea worked, although the effects were strong. But over the next few weeks, Randi began to feel more and more sick. Her energy started to disappear. Her muscles felt weak. Some mornings she had to drag herself out of bed. Sometimes her heart would pound.

When she went to her doctor, he found nothing.

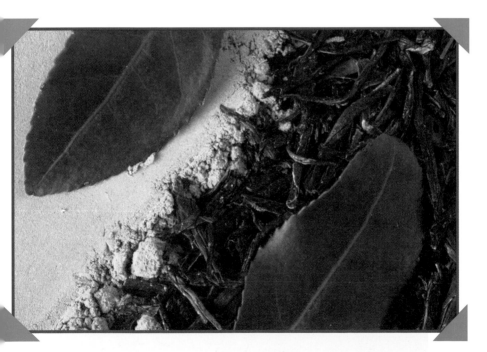

While herbal teas are generally soothing and harmless, it is important to read their labels. Sometimes they may contain ingredients that the user was not aware of.

Medical tests also showed nothing. Meanwhile, she got steadily worse. At this point, she had been drinking the herbal tea for three months. Then Randi's mother suggested that the tea could be causing the health problems. At first, Randi said no. Then she stopped taking it for a day. "The effect was dramatic," Randi remembered. "The next morning I was already feeling much better."[12]

Randi began to research the list of ingredients in the herbal tea. She found that some of the herbs were rather powerful laxatives. These herbs had been dehydrating her body. They also had started to change the balance of minerals in her body. That is what was making her heart pound. Randi sent a report to the FDA. Then she went to local health-food stores. To protect customers, she asked them to stop selling dieter's teas. The stores refused.

four

Dangers of Herbal Remedies

Natural herbs have long been the source of various prescription and over-the-counter medicines. About 25 percent of today's prescription drugs contain ingredients that were originally found in plants.[1]

A Long History

Since recorded history, people have used various plants as medicine. Sumerians, who lived in the Middle East, wrote on clay tablets about plants they found useful. Chinese records from at least 2800 B.C. describe many herbs. Egyptian writings from about 1500 B.C. describe seven hundred plants.

A number of medical books and writings began to appear during the Middle Ages (A.D. 400 to A.D. 1400). These writings usually were recipes, including herbs, for the treatment of common health problem. By the 1500s and 1600s, herbals and "Books of Secrets" provided people with information on do-it-yourself healing.[2] This trend continued into the 1700s and 1800s. By then, some doctors wanted to "popularize medicine and make it part of the general public education."[3]

In 1769, a comprehensive home medical book was published. It was called *Domestic Medicine*. William Buchan, the author, was a doctor in Edinburgh, Scotland. The book sold very well. It was updated and reprinted for many years in America and Great Britain. In his book, Buchan recommended various herbals to treat ill or injured people. Other medical books began to appear regularly in America.

Competing with books like Dr. Buchan's was another type of medical self-help book. These authors said that every person should be his or her own doctor. One of the most popular books was *Primitive Physick* by John Wesley. It was first published in 1747 in London. It was reprinted in Philadelphia, Pennsylvania, in 1764. After that, it was regularly updated until well into the 1800s. Wesley described many diseases, symptoms, and injuries and then gave several treatments. Most treatments were herbal remedies.

Books like these were important. Some people had no access to doctors, especially if they lived in the country or were on a ship at sea. Until the Civil War (1861–1865), some plantation owners used these books to treat their slaves.

For other people, herbal healing was a skilled art learned from a parent or a healer. These people seldom used books. Healers knew what plants helped various health problems. They added to their herbal knowledge through trial and error.

Modern Medicines

In the United States, some people stopped using herbal remedies during the mid- to late-nineteenth century. Scientists had stepped in. They began to find the active ingredients in various herbs. Companies then started to make large amounts of medicines based on these herbs. With the arrival of antibiotics in the 1940s, many herbal remedies fell out of favor. Antibiotics are synthetic, or laboratory-made, drugs that destroy specific bacteria.

A number of modern medicines come from plants. Some examples are listed below.

Pharmaceutical companies have scientifically tested and the The Food and Drug Administration (FDA) has approved all these medicines. In contrast, herbal preparations are not considered medicines. The FDA does not regulate their claims, side effects, or interactions.

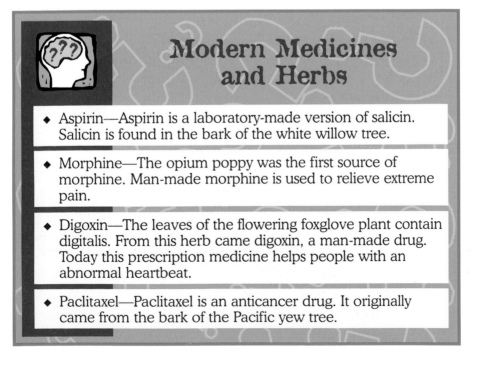

Modern Medicines and Herbs

♦ Aspirin—Aspirin is a laboratory-made version of salicin. Salicin is found in the bark of the white willow tree.

♦ Morphine—The opium poppy was the first source of morphine. Man-made morphine is used to relieve extreme pain.

♦ Digoxin—The leaves of the flowering foxglove plant contain digitalis. From this herb came digoxin, a man-made drug. Today this prescription medicine helps people with an abnormal heartbeat.

♦ Paclitaxel—Paclitaxel is an anticancer drug. It originally came from the bark of the Pacific yew tree.

Companies must make sure their medicines are more predictable and safer than the original herb they came from. For example, a doctor would not recommend that someone with a heart problem chew on foxglove leaves because that could make the heart beat faster. The dosage and effects of the herb would not be predictable.

Herbs Defined

An herb is a plant or plant part valued for its medicinal, savory, or aromatic qualities. Medicinal herbs have real or imagined healing value. Herbs are found among mosses, ferns, trees, shrubs, flowering plants, and even algae. Algae are a large group of plants that lack true roots, stems, and leaves. They grow mostly in water.

Many parts of herbs are used in remedies. Here are examples.

Leaves and Stems

The leaf is the most often used part of an herb.

- *Lemongrass.* The lemon-flavored stems of this grasslike herb are used medicinally, as well as in cooking.
- *Tea.* Tea leaves have been a beverage for thousands of years. Drinking green tea is said to prevent some cancers.

Flowers

Many herbs grow flowers.

- *Silverweed.* This ever-growing plant has yellow flowers. Tea made from the flowers is said to reduce bleeding, swelling, diarrhea, and sore throats.

Seeds, Fruits, and Nuts

Seeds are produced by flowering plants. With the right conditions, seeds can grow into a new plant. Fruit is the fleshy or juicy plant part of a flowering plant. A nut is the fruit or seed with a hard shell. Seeds yield coffee, cocoa, and cola. All three are stimulants and have been used medicinally, for relief from headaches and to increase energy, as well as for flavoring foods and beverages.

- ◆ *Billy Goat Plum*. An Australian fruit that supposedly stimulates the appetite.

Rhizomes

Rhizomes are the underground stems of the ginger plant.

- ◆ *Ginger*. Supposedly reduces nausea, fever, muscle pain, and fatigue.

Bark, Wood, Resin, and Gum

Wood and its top-most layer of bark are found in the trunk, limbs, and roots of trees and shrubs. Resins and

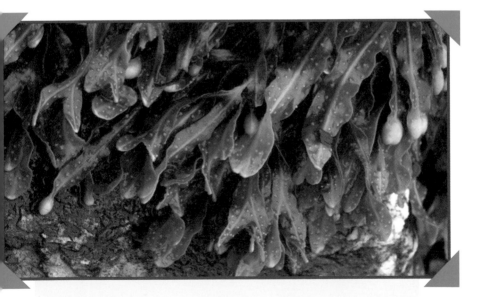

An herb is defined as any plant or part of a plant that is valued for its medicinal, savory, or aromatic qualities. Herbs can be found among trees, shrubs, flowering plants, and even algae (as shown here).

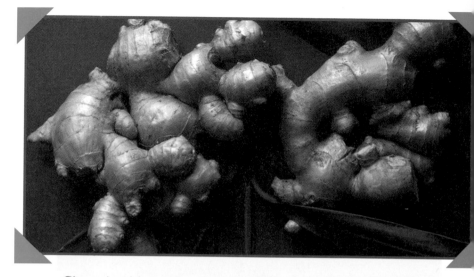

Ginger is said to reduce nausea, fever, muscle pain, and fatigue. Ginger comes from the rhizome (the underground stem) of the ginger plant.

gums are sticky and do not dissolve in water. Trees make them to protect themselves when damaged.

- *Witch hazel.* A shrub with smooth brown bark and fragrant flowers. The leaves and twigs are said to help skin problems.
- *Oriental Sweet Gum tree.* This tree has tiny yellow-green flowers and orange-brown bark. Its bark contains storax, a resin. Storax supposedly helps skin problems.

Essential Oils

The concentrated aromatic essence of herb plants. Oils are found in special cells of the herbs' flower, bark, wood, leaves, stems, and roots. More than four hundred essential oils have been identified.

- *Jasmine.* The essential oil jasmine is said to lift depression and relax people.

◆ *Rose.* The essential oil is supposed to give people energy.

Dietary Supplements Defined

As defined under the Dietary Supplement and Health Education Act (DSHEA), dietary supplements are products that add to the diet. These products include vitamins, minerals, herbs and other plant-derived substances, and amino acids. Amino acids are the individual building blocks of protein.

It is easy to spot a dietary supplement. The DSHEA requires companies to include the words *dietary supplement* on product labels. As of March 1999, a Supplement Facts panel must be on the labels of most dietary supplements.

Herbal and other dietary supplements come in many forms, including tablets, capsules, powders, softgels, gelcaps, oils, creams, ointments, and liquids. They are sold in many places such as health-food, grocery, and drug and national discount chain stores. They are also sold through mail-order catalogs, television programs, the Internet, and direct sales.

What Dietary Supplements Are Not

Dietary supplements, including herbals, are not medicines. It is true that some medicines have been developed from plants. However, a medicine is a substance that can help diagnose, cure, treat, or prevent diseases or conditions. Herbal remedies, by law, cannot make any of these claims. If an herbal remedy is labeled as a treatment or cure for a specific disease, the FDA would consider it unauthorized.

Before drugs can be sold, they must undergo many years of studies. These studies determine their effectiveness, safety, possible interactions with other substances, and dosages. The FDA must review all this information. If the information is sound, then the FDA approves the drugs for sale. Herbal remedies do not go through this process.

Do Herbal Remedies Work?

In 1988, the German government set up Commission E. This group reviews information about herbal remedies. So far, Commission E has published about three hundred papers about popular herbal remedies. This information has been slow to arrive in the United States, however. In addition, the FDA, herbal experts, and makers of herbal products often disagree on the meaning of the Commission E reports.

What does this all mean? According to Dr. Varro E. Tyler, a professor of pharmacy and pharmaceutical sciences at Purdue University, "Practically all [of the literature promoting herbs] recommends large numbers of herbs for treatment based on hearsay, folklore, and tradition. The only criterion that seems to be avoided in these publications is scientific evidence."[4]

The bottom line is that most herbal remedies are untested. Without reliable scientific evidence, no one really knows for sure if most herbals work.

Herbs That May Help

The following list contains herbs that *may* help. Most of these herbs have very little scientific evidence to support their claims. In fact, most have never been scientifically studied in actual experiments with people.

Chamomile
Is used for indigestion. Some research suggests that chamomile tea may help ease discomfort in the digestive tract. But it may cause a bad reaction in people allergic to ragweed or any member of the daisy family. High-quality chamomile smells like apple and uses the whole flower.

Echinacea
Is used to boost immune system. A few studies suggest this herb may help the body fight off infections. However, the effect is only temporary. It may cause a bad reaction in people allergic to any member of the sunflower family. This herb should not be taken by people with diseases such as rheumatoid arthritis and lupus. An alcohol-based

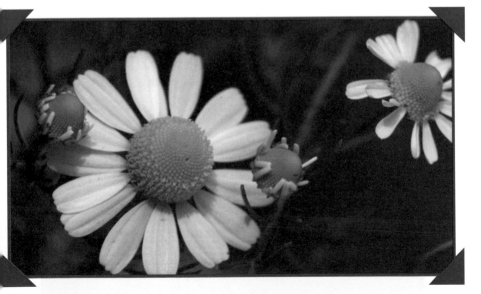

Chamomile, a common ingredient in some herbal teas, is said to help ease discomfort in the digestive tract. Some people, however, may be allergic to chamomile.

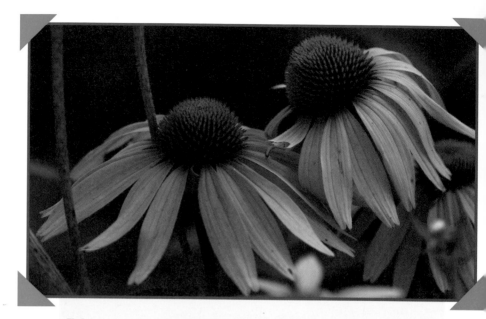

Echinacea is said to help the body fight infections. However, it may cause a bad reaction in people who are allergic to any member of the sunflower family.

solution (liquid) seems more likely to help than capsules. Any possible benefit appears to disappear with continued use of echinacea.

Feverfew

Is used for migraine headaches. Based on one study, it may reduce the occurrence of migraine headaches. Capsules can cause mouth sores. Chewing leaves can cause mouth soreness and lip swelling.

Garlic

Is used for high cholesterol. A couple of studies suggest that garlic may slightly lower cholesterol if taken in large amounts. Too much garlic can stop blood from clotting. People who regularly use aspirin or blood thinners should not take too much garlic. This herb can produce bad breath, body odor, gas, heartburn, and upset stomach.

Ginger
Is used for nausea. Some research may suggest that ginger can prevent motion sickness. However, it may keep the blood from clotting and may cause bleeding problems if taken with certain prescription medications.

Ginkgo biloba
Is used for blood circulation. Several studies suggest that this herb may increase blood flow to the brain and legs. Few side effects have been reported. Some ads say that ginkgo biloba is said to improve memory in healthy people. No study has shown this to be true.

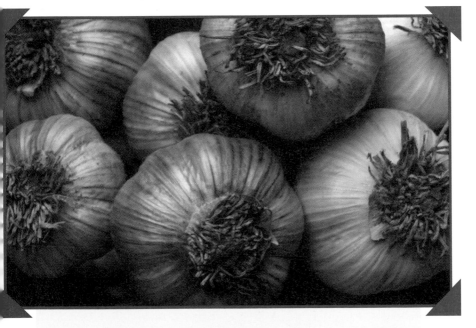

Garlic, a common ingredient in cooking recipes, is said to lower cholesterol levels if it is taken in large amounts. Too much garlic, however, could stop blood from clotting properly.

Saw palmetto

Is used for urinary problems. Several studies suggest this herb can improve urinary flow in men. Saw palmetto's active ingredients do not dissolve in water, so drinking herb tea is not helpful.

Valerian

Is used for sleep problems. Several studies suggest this herb may be mildly relaxing. However, it has caused severe liver damage in some people and can cause daytime drowsiness, lack of coordination, and tiredness. Valerian smells bad, like old socks or sharp cheese.[5]

The information provided about the herbs previously mentioned is not a recommendation to buy and use these herbal remedies. Some of these herbs appear to cause no harm. Others should not be used for regular medical treatment.

What About Other Herbals?

There are more than fourteen hundred other herbs sold to consumers.[6] Most of the makers' claims, though, are unproven.[7] Here is some information on several well-hyped herbal remedies.

St. John's Wort

St. John's Wort sells well in America. This herb is a bush with many yellow flowers. Companies claim it can treat depression. The possible long-term side effects of St. John's Wort have not yet been studied scientifically.[8] Short-term side effects include eye and skin sun sensitivity. Pregnant women and women who are to become pregnant should avoid taking this herb.

Depression is a serious illness. Like cancer or other

serious diseases, depression should not be self-diagnosed. A doctor would know best whether something like St. John's Wort would be helpful.

Ephedra or Ma Huang
Ephedra has been used in China for more than four thousand years. The Chinese have used this herb to treat symptoms of asthma, colds, and flus. Today, ephedra is used in prescription medicines to treat asthma. This herb is also misused by many people as an herbal energy booster.

Companies claim that ephedra is an energy booster that can also stimulate the mind. These claims are not proven. Since 1994, the FDA has received over eight

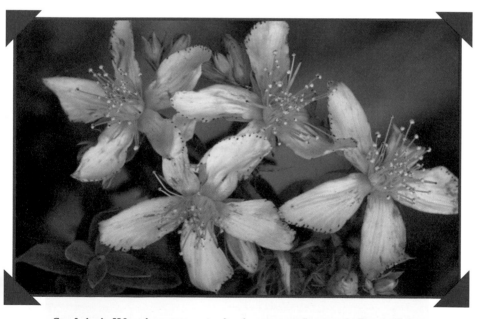

St. John's Wort has come to be known as "nature's Prozac" for its apparent ability to treat mild depression. Short-term side effects include eye and skin sun sensitivity. Long-term effects have not yet been studied scientifically.

hundred reports of negative reactions to ephedra. These reactions have included high blood pressure, sleep problems, nervousness, headaches, seizures, heart attacks, and strokes.[9] At least fifteen people have died.[10] As a result, in June 1997, the FDA proposed guidelines for regulating ephedra. If passed, the regulations would:

- limit the amount of ephedra in dietary supplements;

- require warning labels. The labels would warn people that too much ephedra is dangerous, and not to take ephedra for more than a couple of days.

So far, four states—Florida, Tennessee, Oklahoma, and Louisiana—have stopped all sales of herbal remedies containing ephedra.

Herbal Weight-Loss Remedies

Herbal weight-loss remedies are big business in the United States. According to the Federal Trade Commission (FTC), Americans spend 5 to 6 billion dollars for herbal weight-loss remedies each year.[11] These products appear to be a waste of money. "There's no herb that's been proven to induce [cause] weight loss," said Dr. Varro Tyler.[12]

Usually the herbal product's label does not say how weight loss occurs. But the names of many dieter's teas suggest that the products can promote weight loss. For example, some products use these words in their names: dieter's, diet, trim, slim, fat buster, or fat burning.

Some so-called weight-loss herbs can cause bad cramps, nausea, diarrhea, and a pounding heart. Long-term use of some diet herbs can lead to damage of the colon and heart, and even death. Here are some herbs that claim to cause weight loss.

Ephedra or Ma Huang

Ma huang, a Chinese herb, contains a stimulant called ephedrine. Many herbal diet teas and some remedies contain this herb. Can cause high blood pressure, rapid heartbeat, muscle injury, nerve damage, and death. No proof exists that ephedrine helps people lose weight.

Herbal Fen-Phen

Is *not* similar to the prescription drug combination known as fen-phen. The FDA stopped all sales of prescription fen-phen due to safety concerns. In November 1997 the FDA began to stop the sale of herbal fen-phen products. Chickweed, ginseng, bladder wrack, kelp, licorice, white willow bark, astragalus, burdock, alfalfa, marshmallow, uva-ursi, and horsetail claim to help in weight loss. Some of these herbs can be poisonous in large amounts. No scientific evidence supports the weight-loss claims for these herbs.

Herbal Diet Teas

Some herbs in diet teas can harm the heart and colon. Avoid teas containing comfrey, lobelia, woodruff, tonka beans, melilot, sassafras root, senna, aloe, rhubarb root, buckthorn, cascara, and castor oil. Herbal teas have not been shown to cause weight loss.

Starch Blockers

Promise to block starch digestion. Can cause nausea, vomiting, diarrhea, and stomach pains. The claim of blocking starches is unproved.

Fat Blockers
Claim to physically absorb fat and interfere with the fat a person eats. Fat blockers do not work, and they do not cause weight loss.

Bulk Producers or Fillers
Some bulk producers or fillers may absorb liquid and swell in the stomach. Some fillers are harmful. They can cause blockage in the intestines, stomach, or esophagus. The FDA has stopped sales of these products. Some bulk producers or fillers may reduce hunger, but only for a short time.

Ergogenic Aids
Ergogenic means the potential to increase work output. So-called ergogenic aids promise to pump up muscles, speed metabolism, and cause weight loss. Hundreds of ergogenic aids are sold, including various herbs such as guarana. There is no scientific evidence that they work.

In March 1997, the FTC started Operation Waistline. This campaign warns people of the dangers and false claims of herbal and other dietary supplements.

five

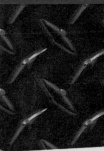

Things to Watch For

This chapter offers practical advice about buying and using herbal remedies.

Beware

Herbs may seem harmless. Ads and claims often talk about the power of herbs. Herbs can be as strong as prescribed medicines, but they can also be dangerous. Here is how to use herbal remedies safely.

Buying Herbal Remedies

- ◆ Buy only herbals whose labels identify the plants and explain when not to use the herb.

- ◆ Stick with a reliable brand. Because herbal remedies are unregulated, their strength may vary. Switching brands can lead to side

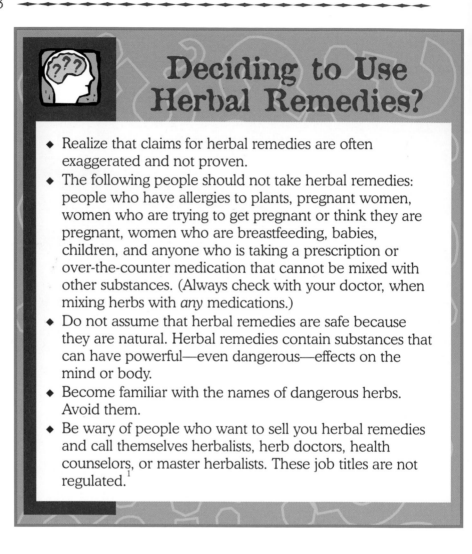

Deciding to Use Herbal Remedies?

- Realize that claims for herbal remedies are often exaggerated and not proven.
- The following people should not take herbal remedies: people who have allergies to plants, pregnant women, women who are trying to get pregnant or think they are pregnant, women who are breastfeeding, babies, children, and anyone who is taking a prescription or over-the-counter medication that cannot be mixed with other substances. (Always check with your doctor, when mixing herbs with *any* medications.)
- Do not assume that herbal remedies are safe because they are natural. Herbal remedies contain substances that can have powerful—even dangerous—effects on the mind or body.
- Become familiar with the names of dangerous herbs. Avoid them.
- Be wary of people who want to sell you herbal remedies and call themselves herbalists, herb doctors, health counselors, or master herbalists. These job titles are not regulated.[1]

effects because each brand may have different potency.

- Herbal extracts are much stronger than whole herbs. Check to see what is on the label.

- Look for accurate information about herbal remedies.

- Avoid herbal remedies sold for a lot less than

competing brands. The company probably has substituted all or part of the herb with an inferior, cheaper ingredient.

♦ Look for ingredients in products with a U.S.P. (United States Pharmacopeia) notation. This means the company followed controlled standards.[2]

Look for herbal remedies made by nationally known food and drug makers. These products are more likely to have been made under tight quality controls. These companies already hold to manufacturing standards for their other products.

Write to the herbal remedy company for more information. Ask the company about the conditions under which its products were made.

Taking Herbal Remedies

♦ Before you take any herbal remedy, read the label.

♦ Do not take any herbal remedy for more than a few days.

♦ Taking more than the recommended dose can cause problems. Use only what the label recommends.

♦ If taking an herbal remedy, tell your doctor.

♦ If an herbal product seems to cause any problems, stop taking it. Tell your doctor of side effects, such as diarrhea, rash, nausea, and stomach pains.[3]

Problem Herbs

Perhaps the most dangerous misinformation occurs when an herb's benefits are given, but nothing is said about its side effects. The FDA has identified a number of herbs that can cause serious harm.

Popular Herbs and Possible Dangers

Chamomile
One of the world's most widely used herbs. Used for upset stomach. Can cause allergic reactions such as itchy skin or rashes in some people.

Chaparral
A traditional American Indian medicine. Promoted as a blood purifier, acne treatment, and cancer cure. Has caused serious, possibly irreversible, liver damage. Still being sold under various brand names.

Comfrey
Used to treat sprains and problems of the lung and skin. Available in many forms: tea, tablet, capsule, lotions. Roots and leaves contain a poison and has caused liver disease and at least one death. Still being sold under various brand names. Cannot be sold in Australia, Canada, Germany, and Great Britain.

Dieter's Teas
Claim to be a weight-loss remedy, but do not work. Nausea, diarrhea, vomiting, stomach cramps, constipation, fainting, and death are possible.

Ephedra (also known as Ma Huang and Chinese Ephedra)
Used to treat asthma, colds, arthritis. Several states limit or have stopped sales of ephedra. Side effects range from high blood pressure, irregular heartbeat, nerve damage, injury, insomnia, tremors, and headaches to seizures, heart attack, stroke, and death.

Germander
Claims to be an energy booster. Was used for gout, a type of arthritis. Can cause liver disease, possibly leading to death.

Licorice
Used to flavor medicine, throat lozenges, tobacco products, and herbal remedies. Side effects range from headache, tiredness, high blood pressure, water and

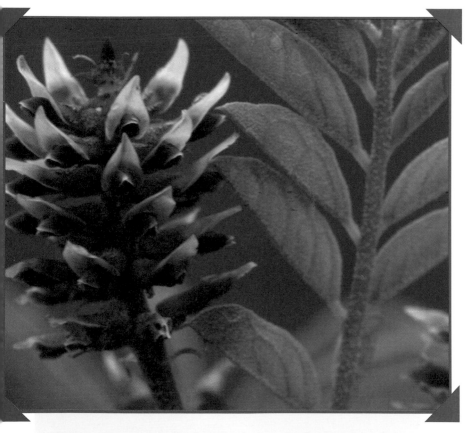

Licorice, a common flavor of candies, is also used to flavor medications, throat drops, tobacco products, and herbal remedies. Possible dangers from overuse range from headache and tiredness to heart failure and even death.

sodium retention to heart failure and death when taken in excess.

Lobelia, also known as Indian Tobacco

Used to treat breathing problems. Acts somewhat like tobacco, but it is not as strong. Low doses cause breathing problems. Higher doses can cause sweating, rapid heartbeat, low blood pressure, and possibly coma and death.

Willow bark

Willow bark is marketed as an aspirin-free product. But it contains an ingredient that changes to the same active ingredient in aspirin. Can cause Reye's syndrome, a possible fatal disease for children with chicken pox, or it can cause flulike symptoms in those who take it.

Wormwood

Supposed antidote for poisoning and a pain killer. Declared unsafe by the FDA. Known to cause numbness of legs and arms, paralysis, weakness, skin rash, and swelling of the arms and legs. Can damage the brain if taken in excess.

Yohimbe

Comes from the bark of an African tree. Supposed to lower blood pressure, reduce chest pains, and treat impotence. Georgia has limited the sale of yohimbe to prescription only. This herb can cause weakness, paralysis, fatigue, stomach problems, and even death.

Fake Products

People need to be on the lookout for fake herbal remedies. These are products that:

- do not do what they say they can, or;

- do not contain what they say they contain; and

- at the very least, they waste people's money. They may also cause physical harm.[4]

Always be wary of claims that sound too good to be true. Chances are, the claims are false or unproved. It is rather easy to spot fake herbal remedies. You are probably looking at a phony product if you see or hear ads, claims, or testimonials (one person's story) that use any of the following words:

Watch for These Words!

- ancient

- breakthrough (there are extremely few medical breakthroughs. Examples of real breakthroughs are the polio vaccine and the discovery of penicillin.)

- detoxify

- easy

- effortless

- energize

- exclusive

- exotic

- guaranteed

- miraculous, miracle

- magical, magic

- mysterious, mystery

- new discovery

◆ purify

◆ secret

Health Information on the Internet

Health is a subject that is covered extensively on the Internet. Over ten thousand health-related Web sites are maintained on the Internet by government agencies, universities, nonprofit organizations, and businesses, and that number is increasing every day.[5] Thousands more online support communities focus on specific health conditions. Online support communities include Usenet groups and electronic mailing lists.

More than 27 million people search for health information on the Internet.[6] With that many people, online marketing and sales of herbal products are growing fast. However, laws for Internet marketing and sales are not well defined, and online information changes quickly. These factors make it difficult for the

BE WARY!

If a company claims that its herbal remedy	Then the product may be fake. Here is why:
Can cure or treat a wide range of unrelated diseases.	No one product can cure or treat many different diseases and conditions.
Is backed by scientific studies, but does not list references or its references are not adequate.	Reliable companies list the scientific studies that back their claims.
Has only benefits and no side effects.	Products that are strong enough to help people are generally strong enough to cause side effects in some people.

Federal Trade Commission (FTC) to try to regulate, or control, online content of ads. The FTC oversees advertising of herbal supplements. To determine if a Web site provides sound information, ask the following questions.

Questions to ask about health-related Web sites

Who maintains the site?
Government, university, and hospital-run sites are usually the best sources for solid health information. Since businesses are usually the ones selling their products, Web sites maintained by specific businesses could be biased.

Does the site focus on a specific product?
If so, this site may be maintained by a business that wants you to buy its product. Be sure to question any information that sounds too good to be true.

Are the names and credentials of the people who prepared and reviewed the site's contents listed?
If yes, you should be able to contact these people by phone or e-mail if you have questions.

Does the site link to other reliable sources of health information?
Government, university, and hospital-run sites usually provide links to other reliable health information.

Does the site charge a fee?
Many reliable health sites offer free access and materials. If a site charges a fee, does it offer value for your money?

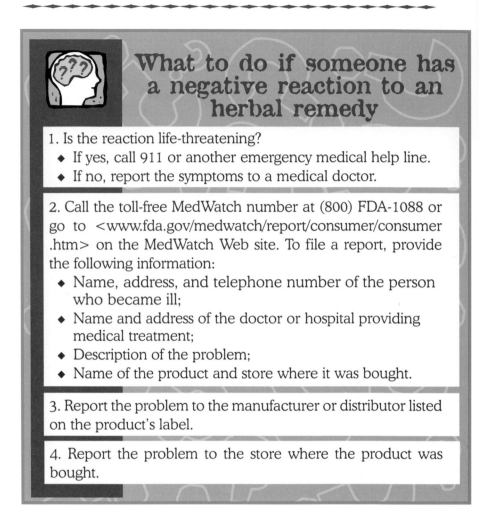

What to do if someone has a negative reaction to an herbal remedy

1. Is the reaction life-threatening?
- If yes, call 911 or another emergency medical help line.
- If no, report the symptoms to a medical doctor.

2. Call the toll-free MedWatch number at (800) FDA-1088 or go to <www.fda.gov/medwatch/report/consumer/consumer .htm> on the MedWatch Web site. To file a report, provide the following information:
- Name, address, and telephone number of the person who became ill;
- Name and address of the doctor or hospital providing medical treatment;
- Description of the problem;
- Name of the product and store where it was bought.

3. Report the problem to the manufacturer or distributor listed on the product's label.

4. Report the problem to the store where the product was bought.

Handling Phony Ads or Internet Fraud

If you find phony herbal ads or herbal-remedy fraud on the Internet, report this to:

- The Federal Trade Commission's National Fraud Information Center (NFIC) at (800) 876-7060; Web site: <http://www.fraud.org>, or send e-mail to: nfic@internetmci.com;

- The Food and Drug Administration (FDA) e-mail address: otcfraud@cder.fda.gov.

questions for discussion

1. Before reading this book, did you know the dangers of using herbal remedies?

2. Do you know anyone who uses herbal remedies? How do you feel about their use?

3. Why do some teens use herbals to get high?

4. The next time you watch television, keep track of how many herbal ads you see. Are you surprised by the number? What types of products are being advertised?

5. What would be three or four things you would tell a friend who asked you about herbal remedies?

6. If a friend or relative wanted to try a herbal tea for weight loss, what advice would you offer?

7. There are many ways to deal with feeling tired besides using herbals or over-the-counter medications. What are three nonpill remedies?

8. Why are herbal remedies accepted more readily in Europe than in the United States?

9. If you could talk to the FDA about better controlling the dangers of herbal remedies, what would you say?

chapter notes

Chapter 1. Pete's Story

1. Geoffrey Cowley, "Herbal Warning," *Newsweek*, May 6, 1996, p. 61.

2. Ibid.

3. Ibid.

4. Ibid., p. 62.

Chapter 2. Social Issues

1. Paula Kurtzweil, "An FDA Guide to Dietary Supplements," *FDA Consumer*, September/October 1998, <http://www.fda.gov/fdac/features/1998/598_guid.html> (May 5, 1999).

2. Lise Alschuler et al., "Herbal Medicine: What Works, What's Safe," *Patient Care*, October 15, 1997, pp. 49–60.

3. Ibid.

4. Ibid.

5. Ibid.

6. J. Harper Liu, "Herbals Go Global," *Transpacific*, March 1994, pp. 28–33.

7. Ibid., pp. 22–24.

8. Barbara Klink, "Alternative Medicines: Is Natural Really Better?" *Drug Topics*, June 2, 1997, pp. 99–100.

9. John S. Williamson and Christy M. Wyandt, "Herbal Therapies: The Facts and the Fiction," *Drug Topics*, August 4, 1997, p. 78.

10. Liu, pp. 28–33.

11. Paul Klebnikov and Zina Moukheiber, "A Healthy Business," *Forbes*, September 21, 1998, pp. 89–91.

12. "Time for a Second Opinion," *Harvard Health Letter*, November 1997, pp. 1–3.

13. Amy Barrett, "Hot War Over Herbal Remedies," *Business Week*, June 8, 1998, p. 44.

14. Dafna W. Gordon et al., "Chaparral Ingestion: The Broadening Spectrum of Liver Injury Caused by Herbal Medications," *JAMA, The Journal of the American Medical Association*, February 8, 1995, pp. 489–490.

15. Sean Mehegan, "Herbal Remedies Promise Drug Firms a Rose Garden," *Brandweek*, October 14, 1996, pp. 32–36.

16. Kurtzweil, <http://www.fda.gov/fdac/features/1998/598_guid.html>.

17. "Consumer Beware," *National Psoriasis Foundation Bulletin*, May/June 1998, p. 10.

18. Mehegan, pp. 32–36.

19. Ibid.

20. Susan Okie, "Looking for Mr. GoodPill," *The Washington Post*, November 25, 1997, p. T11.

21. "Herbal Roulette," *Consumer Reports*, November 1995, p. 704.

22. Ibid.

23. Ibid.

24. Ibid., p. 699.

25. Ibid., p. 702.

26. Ruth Mayer, "The Problem with Herbal Remedies," *Parenting*, May 1996, p. 56.

27. "Herbal Roulette," p. 700.

28. Williamson and Wyandt, p. 79.

Chapter 3. Real-Life Examples of Herbal Abuse

1. Linda Marsa, "If It's on the Shelf, It's Safe . . . Right?" *Good Housekeeping*, April 1998, p. 115.

2. Ibid., p. 116.

3. Susan Miller, "Highs and Lows of Herbal Ecstacy," *Newsweek*, November 6, 1995, p. 67.

4. Ibid.

5. Tony Frasca, Allan S. Brett, and Sun D. Yoo, "Mandrake Toxicity: A Case of Mistaken Identity," *Archives of Internal Medicine*, September 22, 1997, p. 2007.

6. Ibid.

7. Ibid., pp. 2008–2009.

8. Ibid., p. 2009.

9. Judith Mandelbaum-Schmid, "Natural Remedies," *Self*, September 1996, p. 206.

10. Ibid.

11. Ibid.

12. Ibid.

Chapter 4. Dangers of Herbal Remedies

1. Carolyn Kresse Murray, "Cultivating Your Knowledge About Herbal Remedies," *Nursing*, December 1996, pp. 58–59.

2. Guenter B. Risse, "Introduction," *Medicine Without Doctors*, ed. Guenter B. Risse, Ronald L. Numbers, and Judith Walzer Leavitt (New York: Science History Publications, 1977), p. 1.

3. Ibid.

4. "Are Herbal Remedies Good Medicine?" *Consumer Reports on Health*, April 1995, p. 44.

5. "Herbal Roulette," *Consumer Reports*, November 1995, p. 701; Gordon Slovut, "Researchers Give Herbal Drugs Mixed Reviews," *Star Tribune*, (Minneapolis, Minn.), April 8, 1998, p. E3.

6. Ellis Q. Youngkin and Debra S. Israel, "A Review and Critique of Common Herbal Alternative Therapies," *The Nurse Practitioner*, October 1996, pp. 39–52.

7. Ibid.

8. "FDA Warns Against Drug Promotion of 'Herbal Fen-Phen'" *FDA Press Release*, November 6, 1997.

9. Ibid.

10. Ibid.

11. Laura Fraser, "The Herbal Weight-Loss Scam," *Good Housekeeping*, February 1998, p. 103.

12. Ibid.

Chapter 5. Things to Watch For

1. National Council Against Health Fraud, "NCAHF Position Paper on Over-the-Counter Herbal Remedies," *NCAHF Newsletter*, July–August 1995, pp. 2–3.

2. Ibid.

3. Ibid.

4. James H. Lerner, "Herbal Therapy: There Are Risks," *RN*, August 1997, pp. 53–54; Paula Kurtzweil, "An FDA Guide to Dietary Supplements," *FDA Consumer*, September/October 1998, <http://www.fda.gov/fdac/features/1998/598_guid.html> (May 5, 1999); "Herbal Roulette," *Consumer Reports*, November 1995, pp. 700–701.

5. Judy Monroe, "The Net: A Treasure Trove of Health Info?" *Current Health 2*, February 1997, p. 30–31.

6. "Consumer Beware," *National Psoriasis Foundation Bulletin*, May/June 1998, p. 10.

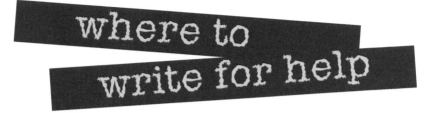
where to write for help

American Dietetic Association (ADA)
216 W. Jackson Blvd.
Chicago, IL 60606-6995
(312) 899-0040
<http://www.eatright.org>

Center for the Science in the Public Interest (CSPI)
1875 Connecticut Avenue, NW
Suite 300
Washington, DC 20009-5728
(202) 332-9110
<http://www.cspinet.org/>

Federal Trade Commission (FTC)
Public Reference Branch
Room 130
Washington, DC 20580
(202) 326-2222
<http://www.ftc.gov>

Food and Drug Administration (FDA)
Office of Consumer Affairs
HFE-88
Rockville, MD 20857
(800) FDA-4010
<http://www.cfsan.fda.gov>

The National Council Against Health Fraud, Inc. (NCAHF)
P.O. Box 1276
Loma Linda, CA 92354-9983
(909) 824-4690
<http://www.ncahf.org/>

National Institute on Aging (NIA)
NIA Information Center
P.O. Box 8057
Gaithersburg, MD 20898-8057
(800) 222-2225
<http://www.nia/health.htm>

Office of Alternative Medicine
National Institutes of Health
P.O. Box 8218
Silver Spring, MD 20907-8218
(888) 644-6226
<http://altmed.od.nih.gov>

glossary

cholesterol—A fatlike substance produced and secreted by the liver, and found in foods of animal origin and in some fat substitutes, such as margarine.

Dietary Supplement and Health Education Act (DSHEA) of 1994—This law created a new category of products—dietary supplements—separate from food or drugs. Herbal remedies are a type of dietary supplement.

hallucinogen—A drug that distorts a person's perceptions. In the United States, laws prohibit the manufacture, distribution, and possession of these drugs except for government research.

herb—A plant or part of a plant valued for its medicinal, savory, or aromatic qualities.

immune system—The body's system that fights off diseases and infections.

laxative—A substance that stimulates bowel movements.

nonprescription—Medicines that can be bought and used without a doctor's supervision.

prescription—A doctor's written instructions describing how to take a specific medication.

side effects—Unwanted, negative, or bad effects.

synthetic—Made from chemicals in a laboratory.

thyroid—A gland in the human body that is located in front of and to both sides of the windpipe. It produces the hormone thyroxine. Thyroxine controls metabolism, or how the body breaks down and uses food.

further reading

FDA Consumer: The Magazine of the U.S. Food and Drug Administration. Superintendent of Documents, Government Printing Office, Washington, D.C.

Fraser, Laura. *Losing It: America's Obsession with Weight and the Industry That Feeds on It.* New York: Dutton, 1997.

Goldish, Mcish. *Dangers of Herbal Stimulants.* New York: Rosen Publishing Group, Inc., 1997.

Hylton, William H., ed. *Rodale's Illustrated Encyclopedia of Herbs.* Emmaus, Pa.: Rodale Press, Inc., 1998.

Thomas, Peggy. *Medicines from Nature.* New York: Twenty-First Century Books, 1997.

index